There were 844 patients included in the study, 752 of which involved open operations, 53 of which involved endovascular repairs and 79 of which were patients who did not undergo operation but received palliative care. It had been hoped to carry out case-mix adjustment for the different groups, but this was not possible because the risk data for those patients admitted as emergencies were missing more often than for those admitted for elective treatment. The overall mortality for open elective operation was 6.2% and for emergency operations it was six times higher at 36%.

The remaining 9% of elective patients were nursed in a dedicated theatre recovery area for an extended period after surgery, though whether this was normal practice in those hospitals, by offering 24 hour recovery facilities or as a result of a shortage of critical care beds is uncertain.

Many of these patients have significant comorbidities, which inevitably require preoperative assessment and treatment, but nevertheless, of those scheduled for elective admission

Abdominal aortic aneurysm is a life threatening condition and once a decision has been made to operate, this should be carried out as expeditiously as possible.

Abdominal aortic aneurysm is a life threatening condition and once a decision has been made to operate, this should be carried out as expeditiously as possible. In patients scheduled for elective major vascular surgery, numerous factors contribute to delays, not least of which is the availability of high dependency and intensive care facilities. Operations are frequently cancelled due to lack of an available critical care bed and the patients in this study were no exception; one in six elective cases having their operation postponed. Not infrequently, the lack of a critical care bed only becomes apparent at the last minute and because AAA repairs are major procedures which occupy several hours operating, large amounts of theatre, surgical and anaesthetic time are wasted with the inevitable knock-on effect on waiting lists. For patients presenting as an emergency, where surgical repair of a ruptured aneurysm is considered life saving, critical care bed availability may be a secondary consideration, but in busy units on major vascular take, for what may be a large catchment area, patients not infrequently spend several hours in the immediate postoperative period waiting for a bed to become free. During this critical time when cardiovascular stability, respiratory function, fluid management, analgesia and temperature control require constant monitoring by experienced staff, such situations are far from ideal.

Of those patients undergoing elective surgical or endovascular repair, 56% went to ICU after treatment and 34% went to HDU.

21% spent more than 12 weeks on the waiting list and 18 patients admitted as an emergency had been on the waiting list for elective repair. Since morbidity increases with increasing aneurysm size and still further with intraluminal leaking or rupture, there is often a fine line to be drawn between optimising a patient's clinical condition in terms of cardiorespiratory system and delaying surgery beyond a certain time.

Vascular surgery is a sub-specialty in which close co-operation and team work between surgeon and anaesthetist is essential to ensure optimal management and patient outcome and this was certainly confirmed by this study. There was excellent consultant involvement in both elective and emergency cases (97% for both anaesthetists and surgeons in elective cases), which is undoubtedly a key factor in the high quality of care delivered to these patients.

Inevitably, a number of hospitals and clinicians were performing very small numbers of AAA repairs, particularly as emergencies, with only 57% of hospitals having an on-call rota for vascular surgery and only 3% reporting an on-call rota for vascular anaesthesia. While the published evidence shows that the outcome of elective AAA repair is better when hospitals and surgeons are performing large numbers of cases and therefore, ideally, this is not the operation for the occasional practitioner, the situation, particularly for emergency cases, is far from satisfactory in many parts of England, Wales and Northern Ireland. This is often simply related to isolated hospitals, where the risks of transferring an acutely ill patient (and usually the only method of transport is by road) with a leaking or ruptured aneurysm are considered greater than operative treatment by a general surgeon in the isolated hospital. The situation is changing nationally, in that, while many of the more senior general surgeons based in district general hospitals certainly have had vascular surgical training and therefore possess the necessary skills and experience, younger surgeons are frequently highly specialised in more limited surgical areas. Few of us would wish to be the isolated surgeon confronted by a major vascular problem which in his and the anaesthetist's view, is unfit for transfer.

Encouragingly, the patients in this study who were transferred did not do worse than patients directly admitted to the operating hospital. However, they are a selected group considered fit for transfer and who survived that transfer. It is difficult to be sure for an individual patient that transfer produces better results than staying put, since considerable additional risk and morbidity can result from delay and transfer, before the benefits of treatment in a specialised unit are realised. Every case is different and factors to be considered include comorbidity, the transfer distance and time and the mode of transport. Equally the benefit of the unit in which surgery will be undertaken is as much about supporting facilities such as critical care provision, haemodialysis etc., as about surgery. Although a surgeon may be geographically isolated, many of the other available facilities may be as good as or better than those available at a tertiary centre, particularly if postoperative critical care facilities in the receiving hospital are severely stretched or unavailable. Many small hospitals still undertake significant numbers of similar cases involving substantial blood loss and rapid transfusion in seriously ill patients. Some tertiary units now run a dedicated on-call outreach service; this team may prefer to travel to the isolated hospital rather than subject a critically ill and cardiovascularly unstable patient to a prolonged transfer in far from optimal conditions. Solutions for improving the service for patients with AAA may therefore differ between geographical areas.

In the case of elective AAA treatment, the well-recognised problem of low case numbers is more relevant and referral or transfer is normally in the patient's best interests. There is little to support surgeons continuing to treat single figure numbers of elective cases on a regular annual basis.

Although the diagnosis and monitoring of abdominal aortic aneurysm by CT scan is widely available and routinely used for elective cases, the availability of specialised imaging services outside normal working hours in many units was considered poor. Whilst in four out of five hospitals that had a CT scanner it was possible to have a CT scan out of hours, only half of all hospitals could organise out of hours angiography or interventional radiography and in only one third was MRI scanning available out of hours. Painful and leaking AAAs are often difficult to confirm in the face of alternative differential diagnoses and this study emphasises that Trusts should ensure the availability of diagnostic radiology services including CT scanners outside normal working hours, for all seriously ill patients. Failure to do so will allow the acute aneurysm to progress to frank leakage or rupture before the diagnosis is apparent, when the outcome for the patient may be considerably worse as a result.

Although a total of 79 patients received palliative care, the question of when not to operate is a very difficult one and a greater proportion of emergency patients were operated on rather than received palliative care in large vascular units, compared to intermediate sized or remote units. This may of course reflect the greater experience and skill of specialist vascular surgeons in large units, but advanced aortic vascular disease is a malignant condition in all but name, rendering the patient terminally ill and this should always be borne in mind. In emergency cases in particular, and in patients with significant cardiorespiratory comorbidity, the decision not to operate, linked to properly considered and administered palliative care, should be considered positively and in full consultation with the patient or his or her advocate.

Although only a small number (53) of patients in this study underwent endovascular repair (EVAR), their good outcome is in accordance with published trials. Of these, only one was ruptured and treated as an emergency, the vast majority were unruptured and asymptomatic. Since successful endovascular stenting requires that the patient is cardiovascularly stable, this method of treatment is limited at present, but increased diagnosis and endovascular treatment of asymptomatic aneurysms will undoubtedly reduce the number which eventually leak or rupture. The results of the recent UK EVAR trials show that in low risk patients (those fit for open repair), endovascular repair is significantly more efficacious in preventing aneurysm-related death than operative repair for four years after operation and therefore should be offered to all patients in this category. In contrast, no survival benefit was demonstrated for EVAR over best medical therapy in patients unfit for EVAR. While this does not mean that no unfit patient should ever be offered EVAR, it does mean that every effort should be made to render unfit patients as fit as possible.

There are many recommendations arising from this report, a number of which are as much about organisation of existing facilities as about transferring or centralising services. Major elective surgery should not be considered or take place unless all essential elements of perioperative care are available. Trusts should take action to improve access to Level 2 beds for patients undergoing elective aortic aneurysm repair so as to reduce the number of operations cancelled and inappropriate use of either recovery area beds or Level 3 beds. In addition, in those units where vascular surgery patients routinely receive postoperative mechanical ventilation, anaesthetic departments and critical care units should review together whether those patients could be managed in a Level 2 high dependency unit.

Clinicians, commissioners and Trusts are encouraged to review whether elective aortic aneurysm surgery should be concentrated in fewer hospitals and to take measures to ensure that surgeons, who do not routinely perform elective vascular surgery, only operate on emergency aortic aneurysms in exceptional circumstances. Equally, isolated surgeons should not be put in

the impossible position of receiving a critically ill patient through the A&E department with no support from an outreach or transfer service and no alternative but to operate. Anaesthetic departments are urged to review the allocation of vascular lists so as to reduce the number of anaesthetists caring for very small volumes of aortic surgery cases.

The perioperative diagnosis and management of AAA and in particular symptomatic and emergency cases, is a major consumer of surgical, anaesthetic, radiological and critical care resources. Inevitably these cases compete with other patients for such facilities and significant advances in the treatment of AAA will have a major impact in this area. While it is vital to ensure optimal care for such severely ill patients, it is also important to try to produce good evidence based data to inform the decision making process in key areas such as the transfer of a critically ill patient with a ruptured aneurysm to a tertiary centre and also to ensure that the decision of whether to opt for surgical, endovascular or palliative care is taken in the best interest of the patient.

Dr. Peter Simpson
Chairman - NCEPOD

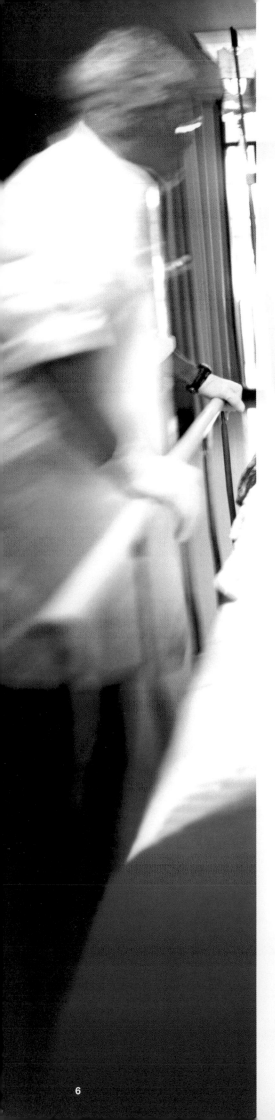

Method

This report describes the process of care of elective (surgical and endovascular repair) and emergency patients with abdominal aortic aneurysms in relation to outcome and also describes the process of care of emergency patients when a decision was made not to operate.

The study was supported by the Vascular Society of Great Britain and Ireland (VSGBI), the Vascular Anaesthetic Society of Great Britain and Ireland (VASGBI) and the Royal College of Radiologists.

Sample size

1,129 operated cases and 106 non-operated cases were expected during the study period. These figures were based on a percentage of the data from Hospital Episode Statistics (HES). An estimate was made for cases from the independent sector.

Data collection

Retrospective data collection took place for two months from 1st February until 31st March 2004.

Hospital participation

All relevant National Health Service hospitals in England, Wales and Northern Ireland were expected to participate, as well as relevant hospitals in the independent sector, public hospitals in the Isle of Man and Guernsey and the Defence Secondary Care Agency.

Population

Data were collected from two groups of patients:

- Adults (≥16 years of age) that underwent surgery for the first time repair of an abdominal aortic aneurysm (AAA); both elective and emergency procedures were included, as well as endovascular repair.

- Adults who were diagnosed with an AAA but did not undergo surgery and subsequently died in hospital during the same hospital episode.

Patients undergoing a repeat repair of an AAA or surgery that was for complications arising from the initial repair of the AAA were excluded.

Questionnaires

A questionnaire was completed by the surgeon that performed the aneurysm repair or made the decision not to operate if the patient did not undergo surgery.

A separate questionnaire was completed by the senior anaesthetist involved.

If endovascular repair of the aneurysm was performed, a supplementary questionnaire was sent to the radiologist involved in the case.

Hospitals were asked to complete an organisational questionnaire relating to the facilities at the hospital.

Quality and confidentiality

Once the questionnaire was complete, the identifying casenote number on each questionnaire was entered into an encryption programme that generated a new unique number for each patient that was not linked to a hospital. The original casenote number was then removed from the questionnaire, along with any identifiable information relevant to the patient or clinician.

Data analysis

The data were aggregated before review by the NCEPOD clinical co-ordinators and advisors.

Analysis of these data has focused on providing descriptive statistical analyses. No attempt has been made to carry out formal statistical hypothesis testing and hence no p-values are presented.

Risk-stratified models of clinical outcome

It had been originally hoped to carry out case-mix correction using a published model [1,2]. Unfortunately, it was found that there was an imbalance in the availability of the data necessary for such risk adjustment, so risk adjustment has not been included.

Advisor group

A multidisciplinary group of advisors reviewed the aggregated data. The group comprised of vascular surgeons, general surgeons who took part in on-call rotas, anaesthetists, intensivists, cardiologists, vascular radiologists, a theatre manager and two lay representatives.

References

1. Prytherch DR, Sirl JS, Weaver PC, Schmidt P, Higgins B, Sutton GL. Towards a national clinical minimum data set for general surgery. Br J Surg 2003; **90(10)**: 1300 – 1305.

2. Vascular Surgical Society of Great Britain and Ireland. National Vascular Database Report. 2002.

Data overview

Hospital participation

226 hospitals were identified as possibly performing surgical or endovascular repair of an abdominal aortic aneurysm.

188 of these hospitals returned an organisational questionnaire.

181 hospitals were eligible to take part in the study. Of these, 163 were NHS hospitals and 18 were independent hospitals.

Of the 181 hospitals identified, 137 completed at least one clinical questionnaire and 21 reported no cases for either month; an 87% participation rate.

Data received

Figure A provides an overview of the number of clinical questionnaires returned. More surgical questionnaires were returned as some of these would have been completed by the admitting consultant when the patient died before being seen by an anaesthetist.

Denominator data

Information on 805 of the expected 1,129 operated cases was received and on 79 of the expected 106 non-operated cases. This represents 71% and 75% respectively.

Population

Figure B demonstrates how the sample population was divided between procedure and admission type.

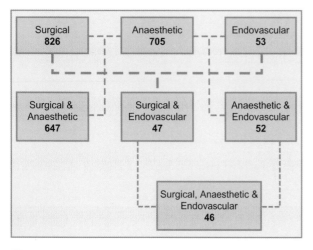

Figure A. Overview of questionnaires returned

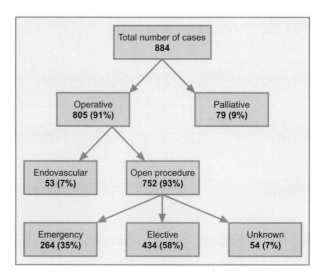

Figure B. An overview of the study sample cases

Organisation of vascular services

Key findings

Imaging

Poor availability of radiology services out of hours was common.

Hospital workload

49 hospitals performed 10 or fewer elective aortic aneurysm repairs in 2002/03.

87 hospitals performed 10 or fewer emergency aortic aneurysm repairs in 2002/03.

Arrangements for emergency cases

Only 57% of hospitals reported that there was a separate on-call rota for vascular surgery.

20% of hospitals did not have dedicated daytime general surgical theatre sessions (NCEPOD lists).

Blood replacement

Only 55% of hospitals routinely provided a cell salvage machine for aortic surgery.

Postoperative care

There was an extensive use of Level 3 ICU care after elective open AAA repair.

9% of patients were reported to have been nursed in recovery areas for a substantial period after surgery.

Outcome

Overall mortality for elective open aortic aneurysm repair was 6.2%.

Overall mortality for open AAA repair after emergency admission was 36%.

Patients admitted as an emergency with an aortic aneurysm were more likely to receive palliative, non-operative treatment in an intermediate sized vascular unit than in a large unit.

Recommendations

Trusts should ensure the availability outside normal working hours of radiology services including CT scanners.

Clinicians, purchasers, Trusts and Strategic Health Authorities should review whether elective aortic aneurysm surgery should be concentrated in fewer hospitals.

Major elective surgery should not take place unless all essential elements of the care package are available.

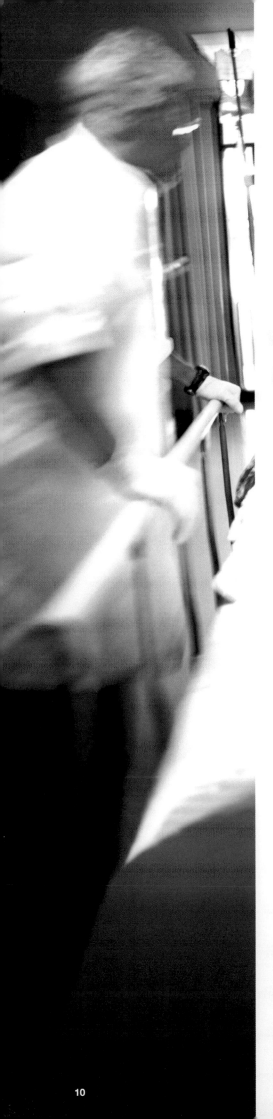

Surgery

Key findings

Waiting lists

21% of patients spent more than 12 weeks on the waiting list for elective AAA repair (Figure C).

18 patients admitted as an emergency had been on the waiting list for either open or endovascular repair.

Cancellation of operations

One in 25 patients had their original operation cancelled because there was no ward bed available.

One in six patients had their original operation cancelled because there was no critical care bed available.

Preoperative assessment

Only 79% of elective patients attended a preoperative assessment clinic.

102 patients were seen by a pre-registration house officer alone or a pre-registration house officer and a nurse practitioner.

The surgeon

In 97% of cases the most senior operating surgeon was a consultant.

All but one of the elective operations for which data were available were performed by a vascular surgeon or a general surgeon with a vascular interest.

92% of these surgeons were members of the Vascular Society of Great Britain and Ireland.

18% of elective patients were operated on by a surgeon who performed fewer than 10 elective AAA repairs a year.

Complications

21% of elective cases had an infective complication of some sort.

1% of patients developed paraplegia.

Emergency operations

19% of emergency admission patients were transferred from other hospitals.

15 emergency operations were performed without a consultant surgeon present.

16 emergency operations were performed by a surgeon without an elective vascular workload.

69% of emergency operations were performed by surgeons who had done five or more emergency AAA repairs in 2002/03.

Recommendations

Patients with an aortic aneurysm requiring surgery must have equal priority with all other patients with serious clinical conditions for diagnosis, investigation and treatment.

Trusts should take action to improve access to Level 2 beds for patients undergoing elective aortic aneurysm repair so as to reduce the number of operations cancelled and inappropriate use of Level 3 beds.

Trusts should ensure that clinicians of the appropriate grade are available to staff preoperative assessment clinics for aortic surgery patients.

Strategic Health Authorities and Trusts should co-operate to ensure that only surgeons with vascular expertise operate on emergency aortic aneurysm patients, apart from exceptional geographical circumstances.

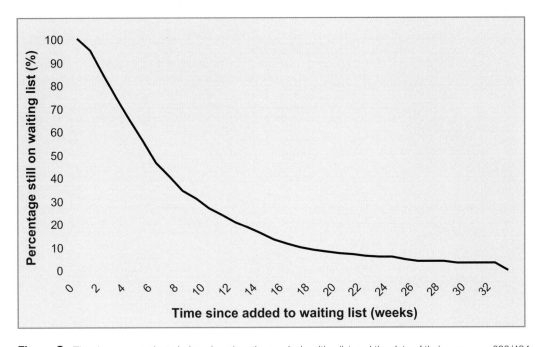

Figure C. Time between patients being placed on the surgical waiting list and the date of their surgery n=382/434

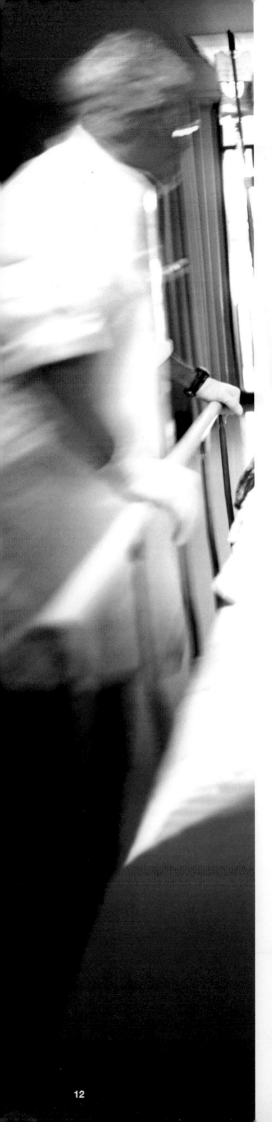

Anaesthesia

Key findings

Preoperative drug therapy

Beta blocking drugs were not widely prescribed before elective operation.

53% of elective admission patients were taking statins at the time of operation.

Preoperative investigations

Echocardiography was the most common cardiac investigation. Other cardiac investigations were not widely used.

22% of elective admission patients were seen preoperatively by a cardiologist.

The anaesthetist

A consultant anaesthetist was involved in 97% of elective cases.

A consultant anaesthetist was involved in 97% of emergency cases.

The anaesthetist was a member of the Vascular Anaesthesia Society of Great Britain and Ireland in 52% of elective admission cases and 26% of emergency admission cases.

Anaesthetic workload

In 49% of cases the anaesthetist could not calculate the number of the anaesthetics they had given for aortic surgery from a logbook or information system.

One in five (22%) elective patients was cared for by anaesthetists who performed five or fewer elective aneurysm repairs in 2002/03.

Three out of five (61%) emergency patients were cared for by anaesthetists who performed five or fewer emergency aneurysm repairs in 2002/03.

Use of epidural analgesia

92% of elective admission patients received an epidural catheter as part of the anaesthetic technique.

In 16% of patients undergoing elective open repair the anaesthetist could not report when the epidural catheter was removed.

Postoperative care

More than half the patients were hypothermic after open surgery.

56% of elective patients went to ICU after operation (Table A).

9% of elective patients were nursed in a recovery area for a significant time after surgery.

42% of elective patients were ventilated after surgery (Table B).

Table A. Immediate destination of patients after elective surgery

Destination	Total	%
Recovery area	35	9
Level 3 care (e.g. ICU)	210	56
Level 2 care (e.g. HDU)	125	33
Level 1 care (vascular surgical ward)	2	<1
Other	2	<1
Died in theatre	3	<1
Sub-total	**377**	
Not answered	57	
Total	**434**	

Table B. Mechanical ventilation of lungs postoperatively						
Ventilation postoperatively	**Elective**	**%**	**Emergency**	**%**	**Not answered**	**Total**
Not ventilated	215	58	42	22	25	**282**
< 4 hours	49	13	9	5	4	**62**
4 – 24 hours	78	21	81	42	11	**170**
> 24 and < 72 hrs	15	4	29	15	3	**47**
> 72 hours	13	4	32	17	7	**52**
Sub-total	**370**		**193**		**50**	613
Unknown	4		6		0	**10**
Not answered	60		65		4	**129**
Total	**434**		**264**		**54**	**752**

Recommendations

Trusts should ensure that anaesthetists can identify the major cases that they have managed in order to support audit and appraisal.

Anaesthetic departments should review the allocation of vascular cases so as to reduce the number of anaesthetists caring for very small volumes of elective and emergency aortic surgery cases.

Trusts should ensure they that they have robust systems for the postoperative care of epidural catheters with accompanying appropriate documentation.

Anaesthetic departments and critical care units should review together whether vascular surgery patients who routinely receive postoperative mechanical ventilation could be managed in a Level 2 high dependency unit breathing spontaneously.